THE PACIFIC NORTHWEST LIFESTYLE

Dylan Jones M.S. RDN, CD, CES

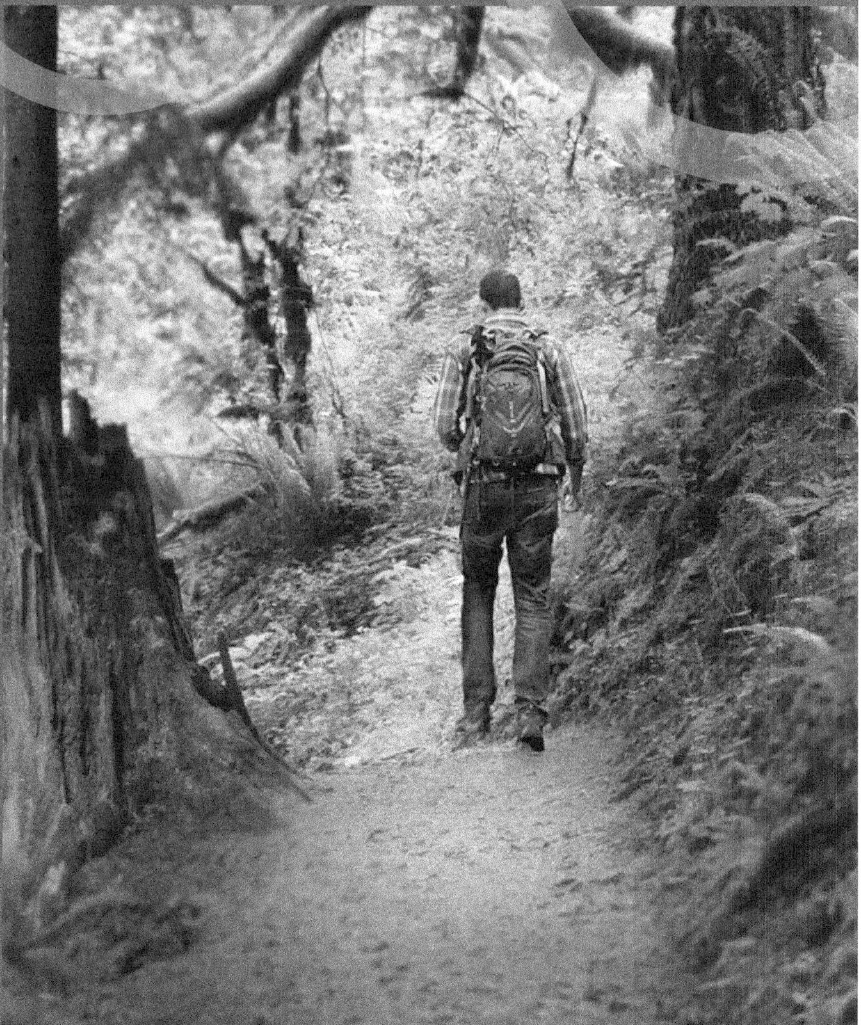

TABLE OF CONTENTS

Chapter 1

WELCOME!

First of all, let me say that this approach I'm about to describe is not my own. It's a borrowed description of the culture emerging throughout the Pacific Northwest area, most notably Oregon, Washington and British Columbia. I wanted to write about the Northwest's approach to health because I sympathize with everyone who has ever thrown their hands up at trying to be healthy, saying "FORGET IT!"

People today are dealing with more misinformation than ever thanks to the latest diet fads. Are carbs good or bad? Should we be eating like cavemen? Is coconut the magic cure —all for every health problem? Then there are followers of all these fads who add to the confusion.... Your friend who swears by Kombucha.... the guy at the gym that says you must take the dozen supplements.... that girl who eats nothing besides bananas and raw, vegan non-GMO kale chips hand-picked in that toxin free country far away.

There's so much confusion regarding our diet and health, and the last thing I want to do is add to this mess of profit-driven, misinforming, awful information that only detracts from people's health. **If nothing else, this guide will illustrate the 5 very most important principles that you can live by to get the largest health bang for your buck.**

The Pacific Northwest Lifestyle is a solution to the misinformation madness, because it describes how some people live much healthier lives without too much additional effort. The people I describe in this book have habits that are enjoyable, their lives are filled with less stress, and they're protected against the common reasons why most Americans (and others) struggle with their weight. Furthermore, it's not a plan that'll require you to count every carb, drink weird concoctions, or follow any other extreme practice.

So with that being said, let's jump into how you can live healthfully like a Pacific Northwest local!

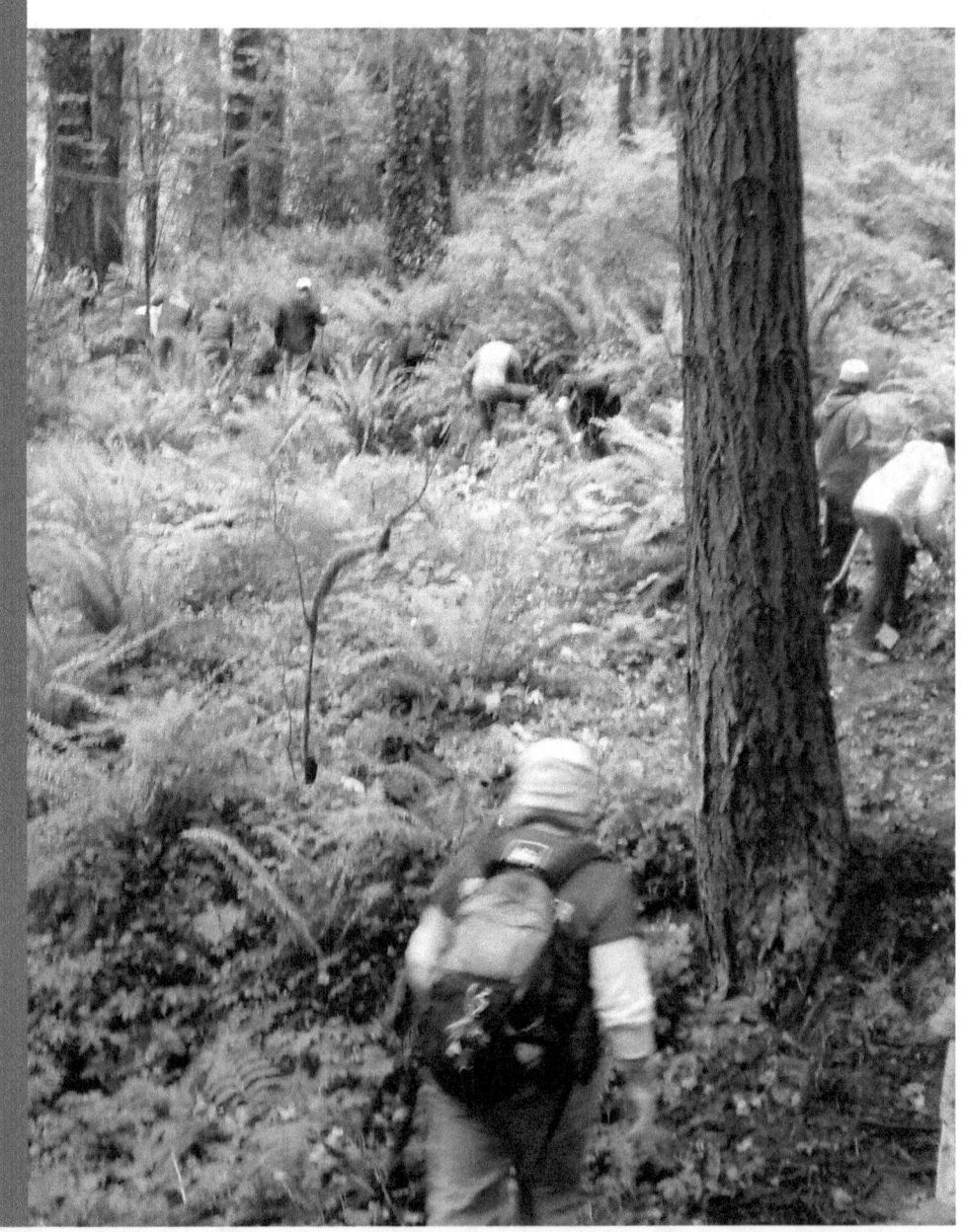

Chapter 2

INTRODUCTION TO THE PACIFIC NORTHWEST LIFESTYLE

This guide will provide solutions for losing weight, gaining energy, managing disease, and so much more, BUT you'll find that the conversation we will have to get to these results is much different than one you've ever had before.

Just like people, our health is complex, and being someone who has dedicated his life to promoting wellbeing and helping others, I'm not about to belittle my readers with a generalized plan that is supposed to miraculously work for every single person. It's based entirely on sound research. This guide will describe the steps that create the greatest health impact and describe why they work. Most people don't have the time to spend endlessly researching the latest scientific

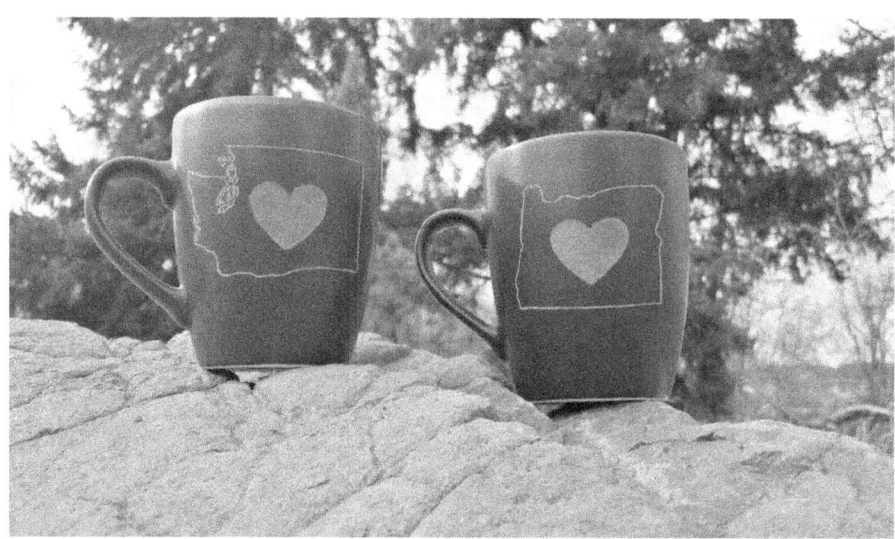

findings on health, so I've done the reading and researching for you, all you have to do is read, learn, and plan using the steps outlined.

In the Pacific Northwest, locals love and cherish the area they call home! It's different, purposefully unique, and those that live here are unconsciously shaped by what surrounds them. Anyone dwelling in this area knows its cultural quirks. It may be unintentional or even unconscious, but many locals are often influenced to ride a bike, shop locally, "chill", eat new foods, go hiking, buy organic, be outside, etc. In short there's a nice plethora of health-promoting habits, seasoned with lively balance.

This brings us to the story behind creating this book. The Pacific Northwest Lifestyle is a laid out observation of what I see as promoting good health in others and what I know medically and nutritionally can work for a great number of other people too! The Pacific Northwest and its locals have many proclivities, both healthy and unhealthy. The lifestyle I'll describe is the batch of healthy ones which seem to make the difference for people in their wellbeing. **It's the nourishing balance of hearty behaviors and not so healthful pleasures.**

Places like Washington, Oregon and British Columbia have some of the lowest rates of the most common diseases. For example, *compared to The United States average, Oregonians and Washingtonians have about half the rate of Heart Disease* (our nation's #1 killer[1]). British Columbia exhibits similar behavior, having just 2.9% reported heart disease in its residents, compared to the country's nationwide 4.8% average [4].

In terms of being physically fit, two of the Northwest's largest hubs, *Portland and Seattle, rank #1 and #3 for fitness in the country*. As I will talk about more in depth later in this book, this isn't due to an abundance of gyms or special sign-up rates at 24 hour fitness clubs...

So why are the residents of places like Washington, Oregon and British Columbia healthier, more fit, and just noticeably different when it comes to health and lifestyle? Some may claim that it's strictly because of a healthier diet or simply because these populations of people are some of the most active. However, I believe such claims really only scratch the surface.

Just like a food cannot be reduced down to its individual nutrients, groups of people cannot be reduced down to their individual behaviors. **There are synergistic effects of living in the Pacific Northwest and it's this unique mix that people use unconsciously and with less effort to live healthier and thrive!**

In all my study and experience with encouraging healthy living, what I keep finding is that truly healthy people don't just eat differently or just exercise more, but that they're also less stressed and rely on basic principles rather than hyped up health fads. Their entire set of mantras is different from those with unhealthy lifestyles.

When it comes to deciding to live a healthier lifestyle, it's a little like smoking. When a smoker decides that they are finally ready to quit the habit and become a non-smoker, they do it not just because they think smoking is bad and may cause cancer, but oftentimes more so because a smoker imagines a life lived to a fuller extent. Without smoking, there are the joys of more energy that allows for a greater experience, better breathing ability, extra spare cash, and more overall freedom to live without needing to satisfy what has previously bound them.

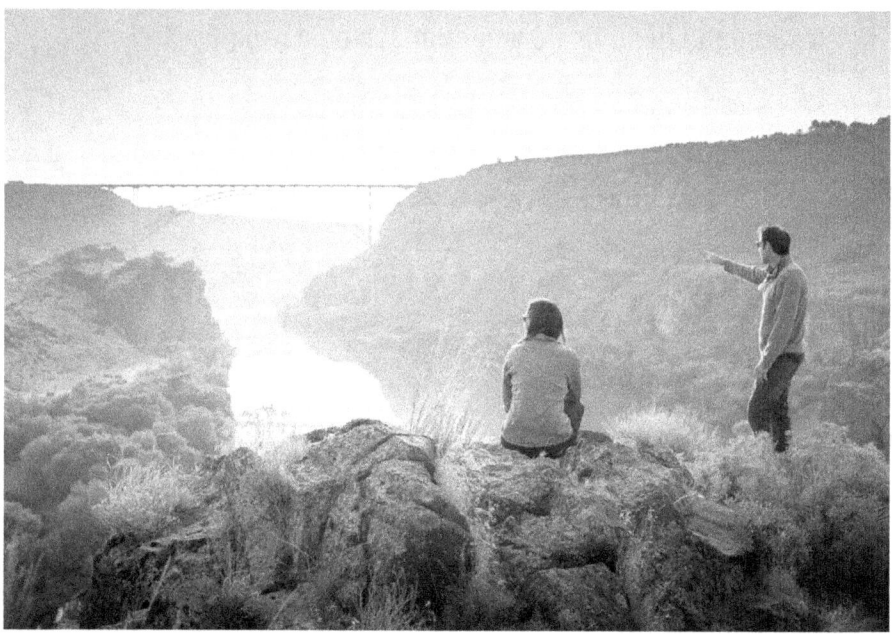

So it goes with living a healthier lifestyle. To correctly spur on grander behavior, it is not about focusing on the fear of consequence from living sub-par health that drives people to be successful, but it is the vision of a superior life with benefits that are meaningful to the individual person. This may mean more energy to accomplish more in a day, the ability to keep up with loved ones, greater self-esteem, extended physical abilities or renowned mental function and mood.

I love to help people answer the individual questions about what foods are good what is bad and what one should do. Everyone one of my answers starts like this, "Well....... *(insert comments about simple principles like having balance, managing stress, activity, etc.)*".

Then, I end with a simple question... "**but why is living healthier really important to you in the first place?**"

I guarantee you that getting asked this question will do monumentally more for you than receiving the answer to your original question!

Lastly, let me tell you this: you don't need to hire me (or anyone else) to ask yourself this question. You can do it right now and get the exact same benefit:

Why is living a healthier life really important for you and what meaningful benefits do you think it would bring?

Your Answer: _____

_____

_____

_____

_____

Possible Examples:

Greater Self-Esteem	Improved Energy	Sleeping Better
Better Mood	Athletic Abilities	Better Libido
Have More Fun	Less Stress of Future	

Chapter 3

THE 5 PRACTICES TO LIVE AS A PACIFIC NORTHWESTERN

#1 Food Has Flavor

As obvious as it sounds, let's go a little deeper into this. Flavor comes in many varities, both healthy and unhealthy. And for ANY plan to work well and be sustainable, food needs to taste GOOD.

Now, the Northwest is known for its variety of foods and unique meals. To live like a local does though, flavor comes from abundant seasoning, savory ingredients, and tasty spices. Let me tell you right now too that you don't have to be a chef to do this effectively. If tiny start-up food carts can whip together delicious dishes in minutes with very little menu variety, you can too! It's about using loads of highly flavorful foods without that don't require cooking for hours that still results in delicious meals.

Here are some of the most Flavor-inducing strategies you can use:

- Sweeten beverages with slices of lemons, limes, and crushed fruit.
- Pack morning smoothies with fresh or frozen berries, as well as chunks of frozen banana.
- Garnish your side dishes with basil, oregano, and rosemary.
- When cooking or warming up soups, lavish them with cumin, garlic, cardamom, and parsley.
- With sweet dishes, mix in spices like ginger, nutmeg, cloves and cinnamon.

- Never have veggies plain! Drizzle them with cold-pressed olive oil, chopped garlic, onion powder, chives, thyme, sea salt, and freshly ground black pepper.

- Dress up salads with red wine and balsamic vinegar or dressings made from creamy tahini, olive oil, or avocado slices.

- For pizzas, rely on roasted red peppers, cooked garlic and savory tomato sauce.

- Sandwiches should have avocado slices or guacamole, onions, and mustards.

- Stir-fries should have cooked bell peppers, artichokes and garlic.

- Lastly, make dips from guacamole, hummus, cashew creams, low fat yogurts, and honey mustards.

Once again, you don't need to be a master chef to put these practices into use. Many of the above ideas can easily be done very quickly and without much culinary experience.

When you've reached the end of this book, I encourage you to look at the "**20 Meals Made with NW Style**" for even more great examples.

#2 Embrace Thy Outdoors

There's something to be said about those who frequently get outside for their recreation. The intentions behind doing it are often so drastically different than those going to the gym or working out at home. This happens to be one of the main characteristics of people in the Northwest. They camp, hike, bike ride, explore, jog, etc. People who do this experience freedom and joy, compared to a gym's sometimes stale and mundane atmosphere.

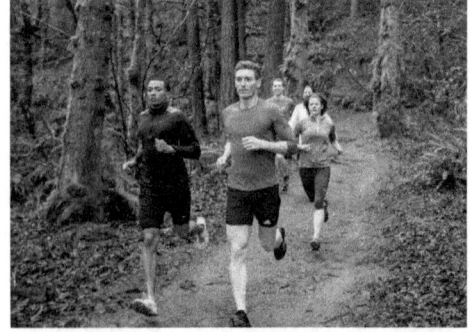

Did you know that there are actually additional health benefits to being active outdoors rather than in gyms? Turns out that research done on outdoor exercise vs indoor shows that people who choose outside exercise get greater feelings of revitalization, feel more energetic, and have larger drops in stress and negative feelings [3].

In a large study of 319 people, researchers actually found that those taking to the outdoors not only felt more restored, but were significantly more likely to be consistent with their exercise compared to those working out in gyms [5]. Furthermore, outdoor environments create greater positive engagement, further decreases in tension, confusion, anger, and depression, and boosts energy [6]. Exercising outside has even been shown to synchronize the circadian rhythm for those who work long hours by balancing hormone levels [7].

Get Outside For Your Exercise, Preferably Daily!

This is a critical part to the Pacific Northwest Lifestyle. The activity of choice is up to you and I'll guide you with some suggestions if you're not so enthusiastic the outdoors. It doesn't have to be much, but it should be on most if not all days of the week and using exercises that are both aerobic and strengthening.

Locally, these are considered "hobbies" - not exercise. Try to adopt the same perception. You can take your pick from any type of exercise including:

Bike Riding	Boat Racing	Geocaching
Hiking	Wakeboarding	Golf
Jogging Swimming	Soccer	Longboarding
Scuba Diving	Street Ball	Gardening
Plyometrics	Bird Watching	Lacrosse
Outdoor Yoga Tai	Camping	Paintballing
Chi	Street Hockey	Kayaking
Baseball	Ultimate Frisbee	Skiing
Rock Climbing	Badminton, Free	Snow Shoeing
Roller Skating	Running	Tubing

The key is to find something fun and enjoyable and do it often. Ask yourself, what can you lose yourself in doing? Is there anything that will help to turn the volume down in life?

You may need to get some used gear to start, or find the right clothing to keep comfortable-but trust me, it's worth it! Outdoor enthusiasts typically have naturally slim bodies and have greater benefits than most indoor gym goers because they're doing what they love and what brings them peace.

If you already know your activity of choice, then commit to embracing it DAILY. HOWEVER, don't be afraid to try new things from time to time. You'll be a happier and healthier person when you do.

Questions to help you get started:

1. Where around you is there a view?
2. Are there nature areas that are easily-accessible?
3. What hobbies or activities do you enjoy?

   If none, find some! Join a group on meetup.com or take a free class offered on Craigslist Events or seek out the local outdoor rec programs offered through your parks and recreation.

4. **Do you prefer a group or to be by yourself?**

   Meetup.com is a great website to find others who are looking to get more active in the local area.

5. **Where is the nearest outdoor park by you?**

   A Small Tip for Staying Active:

   Now, a quick motivation warning when it comes to fitness and remaining active.... if you're simply doing it to look better naked, your motivation is flawed. With changing activity habits (as well as other habits) the reasons fueling your behavior change are going to determine its outcome.

   If you want your activity to stick for the long run, my experience working with clients in the gym tells me that you'll need to find a deeper outcome that is significantly relevant for you. Perhaps you're after greater self-esteem, or need greater daily energy to perform in your life. Bottomline, find something that is deeper than vanity alone.

My hope is that every person can move past the vanity-related reasons that inspire gym sign-ups without gym attendance. You may need to dig a deep hole into your mind, emotions and thought before you find these springs of motivation propelling up and out. Once you do though, it will keep you coming back.

#3 Live Leisurely

Next, we come to the balancing part.

The Northwest is well known for its lavish variety of good drinks; microbrewery beer, local wines, etc. Many people here take pride in the frequent social pleasure of closing a day with one of these enjoyable beverages. This isn't every night, but it's probably noticeably more frequent compared to other places.

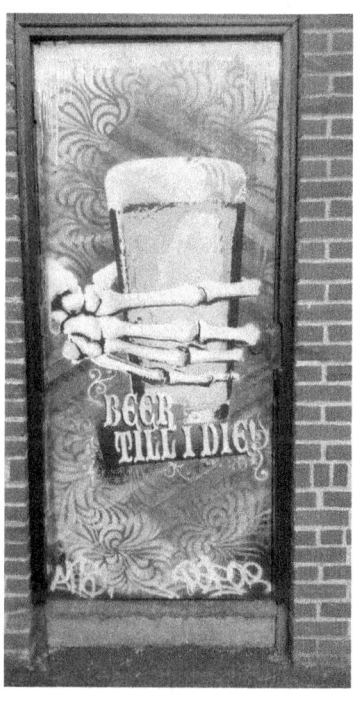

So, is this health promoting? No, not at all! After completing a Masters in Human Nutrition, a Bachelors in Exercise Physiology & Metabolism, becoming a Registered Dietitian and Clinical Exercise Specialist, and working with hundreds of clients both one on one and in groups, do I personally recommend this? Yeah, sure. Let's talk about why.....

Clarifying Alcohol & Health

If you've heard that 1-2 daily alcoholic drinks is good for health, this is a common misconception particular in America.

A large conclusive study clearly showed that given all the damage that alcohol in ANY form does to the body through inflammation and extra calories, in already healthy individ-

uals, there is NO health benefit to ANY amount of beer, wine
and liquor (3).

Many people today live an overly busy lifestyle and the saddest part is that most are oblivious to it. The typical emphasis of American culture is work until you can't anymore and that non-work activities are wasteful.

Now the Northwest uses its snobby drinks for this 3ʳᵈ mantra, but **the real emphasis here is to rejoice daily.** That means putting away work, ideally spending time with others and doing what helps you feel balanced and maintained in life.

This 3rd mantra is just as important as the others, but is also the most likely to become neglected. Psychological wellbeing is SO critical to living a healthy and balanced lifestyle, yet it is almost never practiced. I personally believe that it's a lack of this balance that sets so many up for failure.

James Allen said *"Change of diet will not help a man who will not change his thoughts . When a man makes his thoughts pure, he no longer desires impure foods."*

The point is simple--seek out balance and peace **DAILY.** The local area of Portland and Seattle frequently stop from work to enjoy a beverage and be social or just relax. However, good beer or wine is not required to live a Pacific Northwest Lifestyle, I'm simply pointing out that this is the common practice of balance I have noticed here.

If you can achieve some equipoise through another practice on a daily basis, be it meditation, yoga or something else, go for that. Just make sure it is truly rejuvenating and freeing though, and not just "another daily task" you check off to feel more accomplished or successful.

The key thing here is to remember to relax, enjoy, rejoice, unwind, unplug, sit back, let go, be quiet, take it easy....

(I'm using so many words because I want you to understand how important this is. It's just as vital to a balanced and healthy life-

style, but you'll put it off if you don't realize it. So make this a DAILY commitment!)

Rest, put your feet up, close your eyes, breathe deeply, get composed, sedate, even if it's just for 10 minutes.

Okay, I hope you got it now.

Bottomline, this 3rd mantra is your call to maintain a balanced life through recognizing that psychological wellbeing is just as critical as the activity your body gets or the food you eat.

#4 Mainly a Gatherer, Not a Hunter

Next we come to what I suspect will be the most unfamiliar to most traditional American habits. This is the fact that following the Pacific Northwest Lifestyle is to have a mostly vegetarian diet. This isn't just a common axiom of Northwest citizens though; it's the trait that majority of the world's healthiest cultures follow and benefit from greatly [4].

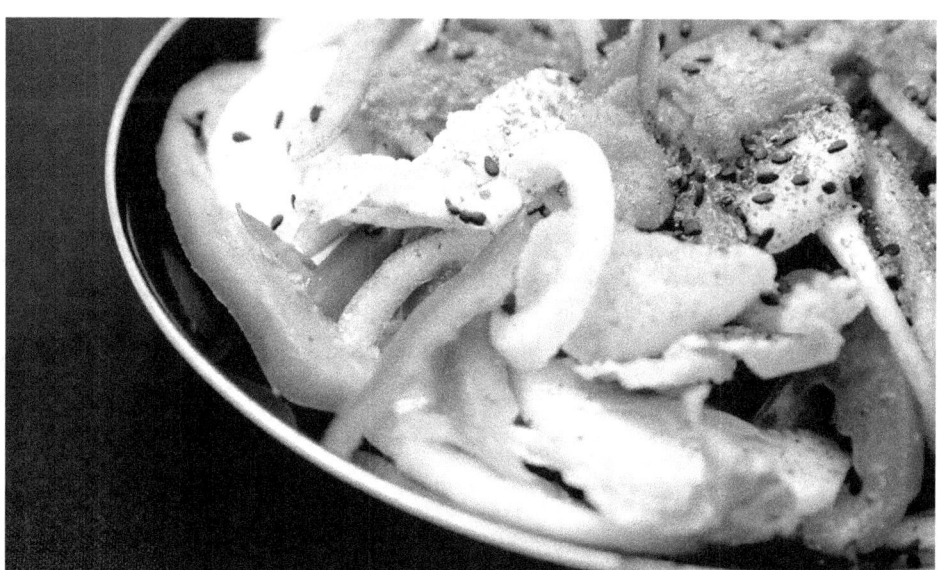

I hope I have not lost you yet. As unfamiliar as this may be for many people, it shouldn't be enough to dissuade you. Having a **"mostly vegetarian diet"** doesn't mean that you never get to eat meat again or that you'll be left with an unsatisfying range of foods. After reading more about this below, I hope you'll see exactly why I've highlighted this as one of the more important practices of living like a Pacific Northwestern.

Like I said, when looking at the habits of the healthiest cultures in the world, a stand out quality is an obvious focus on **more plant foods rather than animal ones**. Take a look below at how this is done in some of the world's healthiest populations:

- *The Japanese Okanowan (oldest living culture on earth) fill their diet with loads of veggies, rice, fruit and legumes. Meat intake isn't forbidden or anything, but it's just saved for special occasions and holidays, so it's a much smaller part of the overall diet.*
- *The original Mediterranean dwellers who cultivated the now popular Mediterranean diet focused on lots of whole grains, fruits, hummus, tons of spices, salads and soups. Meats and seafood were eaten quite seldom.*
- *The Loma Linda Californians who have above average lifespans do totally abstain from dairy and meat, but instead replace it with delicious recipes including lots of nuts, whole grain breads, savory veggie burgers, seeds and large daily large salads.*
- *In Nicoya Penninsula, Costa Rica, abnormally healthy residents focus on eating mainly corn, squash and beans, garnished with a large variety of tropical fruits. Meat is definitely not available enough to eat daily, but that certainly doesn't mean they lack protein or suffer in health because of it.*

So when you look at these so-called "blue zones" (zones with the earth's healthiest populations), you see this same trait repeatedly followed. With it, you also see slimmer waist lines, less overweight adults and most importantly, less disease.

Comparing each of these different vegetarian-esque styles to the typical American diet-which is almost entirely based around animal foods like meat, dairy and eggs-it's no wonder why chronic disease is still on the rise. **The American diet is in direct opposition to how the healthiest populations on the planet live**.

Does a Mostly Vegetarian Diet Lead to Weighing Less?

How does eating more or less meat affect a person's weight? Well, there are two main connections between eating meat and our weight:

1. There is a strong connection between meat and weight, as nutritional studies consistently show that the more meat being eaten, the heavier a person typically weighs. Furthermore, the meat most related to gaining weight is actually poultry such as chicken and turkey [8] (it's also what most people think is the "healthier" option).

2. Also, those eating meat-free diets get higher intakes of nearly every nutrient and typically have a significantly higher resting metabolic rate [11].

Eating meat leads to weight gain even when calories are being controlled. This can be because meats often contain hormones and chemicals that promote weight gain.

> *"Nothing will benefit human health and increase chances of survival of life on Earth as much as the evolution to a vegetarian diet."*
>
> **-Albert Einstein**

All this being said, meat is a very culturally common meal and provides fullness. So how does a person replace meat in their diet? And with what should it be replaced?

Locally in the NW, this trait has been crafted and mastered to be delicious. It's not just about avoiding meat. When done right, it's savory, filling and as enticing as any other style of eating!

I reached out to a couple local restaurants to ask if they could give me a sneak peak of how they keep customers coming in the doors without the typical reliance on meats, dairy, fish and eggs.

—The Bye & Bye Vegan Bar & Restaurant
The Eastern Bowl: Nutritional yeast breaded tofu, broccoli, and brown rice. served with ginger peanut sauce and topped with sesame seeds and avocado.

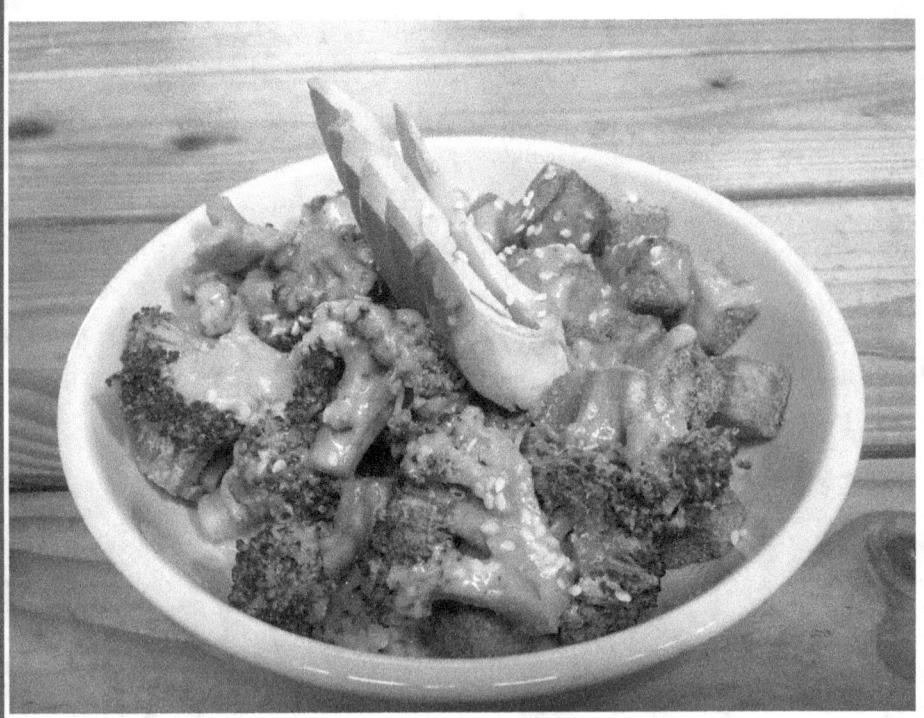

—The Sweet Hereafter Bar (next page)
The Thai: Thai spicy tofu, cabbage, sprouts, carrots, scallions, peanuts, and brown rice.

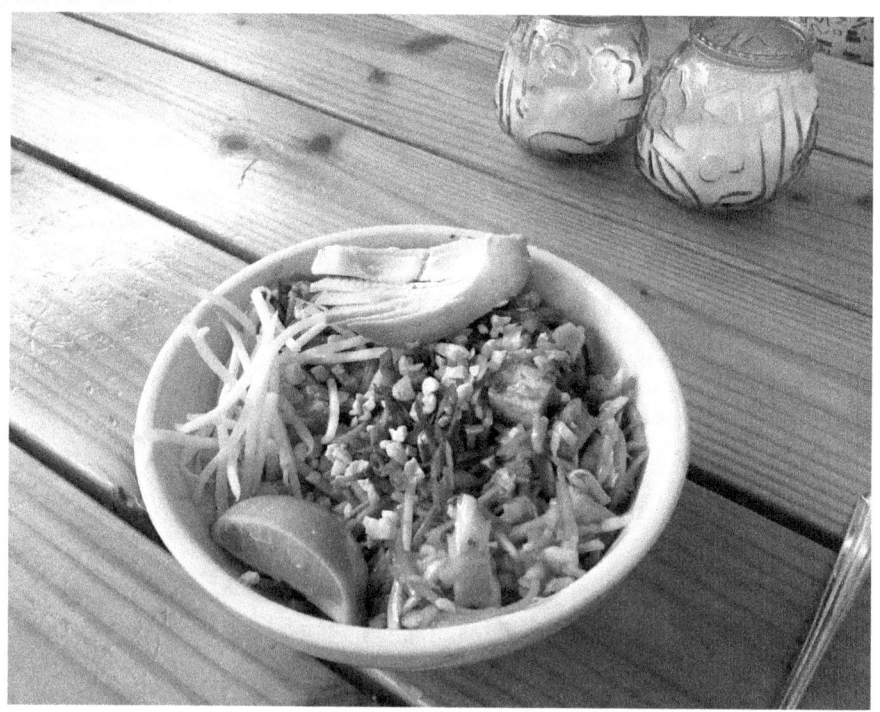

OTHER EXAMPLES:

As someone foraging and following the Pacific Northwest Lifestyle, you can grill up black bean burgers, stir-fry wild mushrooms with onions and garlic, grill kabobs of peppers, zucchini and squash. You can also try marinating seitan or tempeh with BBQ and teriyaki sauces.

Bottomline, mantra #4 must be said because there is almost no other single dietary change which can make such a dramatic difference in a person's overall wellbeing. Research has consistently shown that the individuals who consume a more vegetarian diet than others will result in slimmer bodies, less heart disease, greater longevity….list goes on and on.

Michael Pollan summarizers this practice best. He said **"Eat food (meaning not junk food). Not too much. Mostly plants."**

Pretty counter-cultural right? Nevertheless, when you jump into it fork first using the resources with this book, you'll be shocked at how quickly you'll grow to love the delicious, savory and filling options of this fourth rite of passage to living a Pacific Northwest lifestyle!

#5 Very Little Bags and Boxes

We'll end with just one more precept and hopefully by now there are already enough new thoughts to keep you salivating for more. Thankfully, it's one habit that is now more openly embraced.

This is to have a more "do-it-yourself" attitude when it comes to food. It's to seldom travel into the depths of the middle of the grocery store. In short, **a Pacific Northwest Lifestyle is all about getting food closer to its source**, with little to no processing. Now, many people advocate this, but fail to due to lacking guidance. Let's try to avoid this pitfall. I'll put forth tons of starting examples of this as well as give you *a defining criteria* when you're choosing foods.

*** When following this fifth precept, you'll question what foods in the store really are unprocessed and which ones are merely sneaky food imitators.

There's a solution here that I'll share. I have an adorable little niece who is about 10 years old and once, when eating dinner with my family, I asked her to read me what was listed on the back of a nutrition facts panel. She did pretty well, recognizing most of the ingredients and only stumbling on pronouncing a few. She turned the panel towards me and asked about one saying, "what's sodium benzoate?", to which truthfully I said, "I actually don't really know". So it was then that I decided that a simple safety check for most people would be:

<u>If a food label has words that would confuse</u>
<u>"a 10 year old", don't buy it.</u>

If needed, you can ask the nearest "10 year old" next time you're grocery shopping to confirm with some foods.

So buy food, mostly in whole form. You'll save a ton of money doing this, you'll eat better tasting meals, and most importantly, you'll be saving your health in the process. It's a practice that the Northwest has adopted and nurtured to the fullest extent. The local residents have also adapted this to be a time-saving practice too. I assure you that when done right, following this suggestion gets food from the fridge to your mouth in just as fast of fashion as compared to traditional, processed food methods or compared to relying on fast food for meals.

HOW AN UNPROCESSED EATING PLAN WORKS:

When you're grocery shopping, you must rely on bulk sections for items like:

- Whole grains like quinoa, oats, brown rice and millet
- Nuts and seeds like raw almonds, cashews, walnuts, flaxseeds, sunflower seeds and pumpkin seeds
- Dried fruits like apple slices, dried apricots and dried peaches.

Next, use the produce aisle for the freshest fruits of preference within the budget. Frozen or canned varities are still good and can be a convenient way to fill up the diet too.

Snacking vegetables like carrots, bell peppers, broccoli, grape tomatoes and snap peas come in handy for fast options.

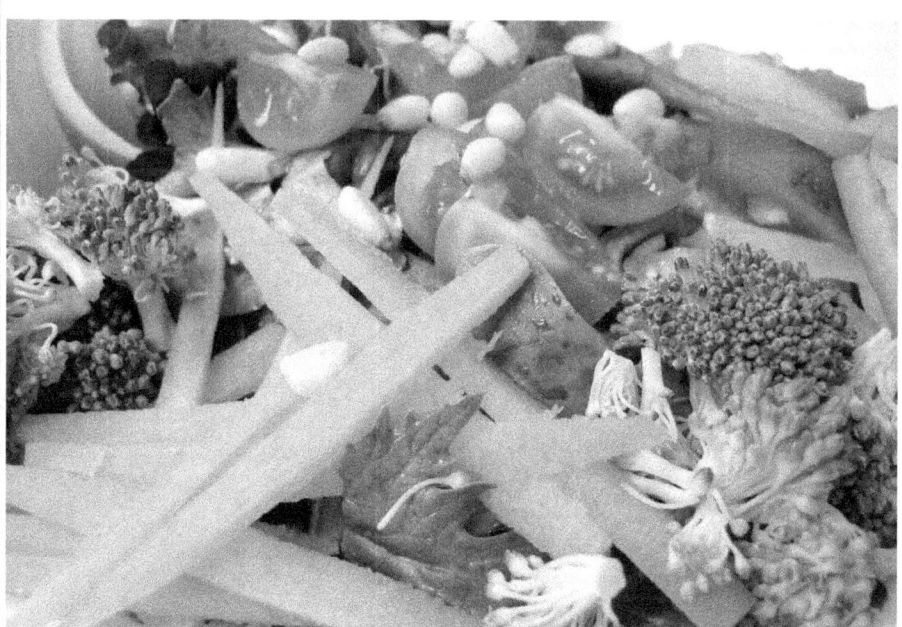

Leafy greens are a critical part to your diet as well. You'll want to have enough to make at least two varities of delicious salads from spinach, red leaf lettuce, kale, green and red cabbage.

Frozen produce is essential (and still VERY healthy) when too busy to prep fresh: Peas, broccoli, brussels sprouts, lima beans, peppers and squash are some of the best choices. These can be quickly microwaved in only minutes for eating. Lastly, relying on frozen forms of berries is a good way to keep them affordable year-round.

A CRITICAL SUGGESTION

A critical part to making this work is having a set aside time once a week to do some basic food preparation. It doesn't have to be long, but I would recommend about one hour per week to do the following:

- Steam or prepare at least five servings of vegetables in quick grabbing containers.
- Use an extra-large pot or crock pot to cook large amounts of any of the following: whole grain, bean or lentil (quinoa, kidney beans, red lentils, chickpeas, brown rice, etc.). Freeze what won't be used in the upcoming week and refrigerate the rest in quick grabbing containers.
- Freeze foods which are prepped so that they can be easily grabbed and prepared in the upcoming week (common examples: bananas, leafy greens, beans, lentils, oatmeal, peas, corn, broccoli, squash, etc.).
- Try to keep your freezer fuller than your refrigerator. Then, move items from the freezer to the refrigerator as they are needed.

Eating food in the unprocessed state is to put on your farmer's hat and act as your own cultivator. By doing this, you are essentially doing the very thing that processed food companies do, yet saving your health and spare cash in the process. It's freeing and gives you a feeling of independence against the cogs of today's traditional processed food trap.

Wendell Berry argues that,

" *To be interested in food but not in food production is clearly absurd.* "

He's right. Take food production back from large food corporations and don't stop experimenting until you've pioneered all your food needs.

For more tips, refer to the Appendix of Recipes and One Week Meal Plan.

Chapter 4

USING THE PAC NW LIFESTYLE TO ACHIEVE A HEALTHY WEIGHT

I expect many people to look through this book for answers related to maintaining a healthy weight. You've come to the right place, as I've helped hundreds of clients with this common goal and know EXACTLY what separates a successful weight loss plan from an unsuccessful one.

—THE LOW DOWN ON LOSING WEIGHT

Losing weight is VERY frustrating and it's understandable that people will do whatever is necessary to get results as soon as possible. Not feeling comfortable in your own skin, having low self-esteem wherever you go and being constantly judged because of your weight-it's crushing. I've seen it completely destroy lives altogether. All of this is for a culturally celebrated belief that you must be thin or look good in a swim suit before being truly happy.

So yes, we all would like to change our bodies right away and we need to do this in a way that doesn't damage our health in the process. An unfortunate part about weight management today is the business side of it. Realize that as someone now looking to lose weight, you are a target for marketers just looking to make a buck with cheap products and ineffective programs.

You've probably heard many things about losing weight which are not true. Advertisers have intentionally spread false knowledge and cite fake research to persuade sales all while confusing the average person. Even worse, many popular weight loss programs today can actually harm health and a person's metabolism when followed, making it extremely important for you to choose the RIGHT plan for losing weight.

WHAT IS THE BEST PLAN FOR LOSING WEIGHT?

The best possible plan is one that emphasizes getting healthier first and weight decreasing in the process. Losing weight and getting healthy…they're two very different focuses.

CAN A PACIFIC NORTHWEST LIFESTYLE PLAN BE FOLLOWED TO LOSE WEIGHT?

ABSOLUTELY! With that said, I have just four extra tips for anyone attempting to achieve a healthy weight while following the Pacific Northwest Lifestyle.

1. Use only sustainable methods

If you're trying to eat a certain diet filled with food you don't enjoy and that you're not satisfied with, <u>IT'S NOT GOING TO WORK!</u>

There are thousands, maybe millions, of people right now trudging through long days of eating no carbohydrate containing food (Atkins), relying on only frozen dinners (Metafast) or drinking disgusting concoctions of lemon juice and cayenne pepper to cleanse. All to *temporarily* shed some pounds which

will no doubt return with "interest". This yo-yo approach to losing weight is emotionally taxing, physically damaging and worst of all, produces no long-term benefits.

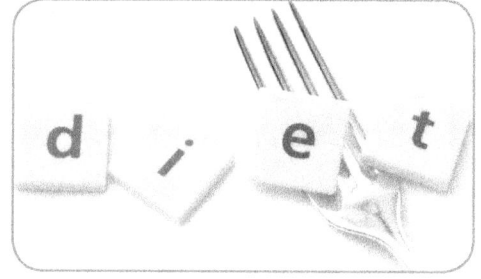

A diet is only effective for as long as you follow it, which is why health professionals today now advocating adopting a new lifestyle. The process of yo-yo dieting and weight fluctuation should be avoided at all costs. I hope you will look to the 5 practices of the Pacific Northwest Lifestyle for an extremely enjoyable way of eating and getting activity.

2. Keep a food log or track your calories.

While this next step may seem tedious, it's also one of the most important. Food tracking is such a critical factor for all successful weight loss plans, shown to help almost everyone in every situation. This may mean using a free phone app to track calories or just simply writing down what you're eating on a daily basis.

This helps us to be more aware of what foods we're intaking, as well as identifying if there are any nutritional imbalances in our diet (lacking nutrients, too much calories, too little, etc.).

If you get burnt out while tracking, no problem! Put it down for a while and then come back when you're ready to.

3. Manage Unnecessary Cues for Eating

Today we live in a very food-saturated and highly stressful environment that can trigger eating at inappropriate times. The large amount of stress in American culture can consistently play into eating behaviors and even lead to long-term disordered eating.

The first step here is to remove tempting treats from your home and work environment. Even, the most motivated person in the world is bound to mess up when constantly in an environment of temptation. A treat is fine every now and then, but let it be on your schedule and when you want it rather than sporadically without notice.

Also, one of the best strategies for management of stress eating is to keep a journal recording emotions and thoughts. It doesn't have to be much, as just 5 minutes of writing how you feel can bring significant clarity and relief.

If you just can't use the writing method, start doing daily meditation (even just 10 minutes). This is like massaging your mind and cultures across the world have practiced this for centuries for its medicinal effects on thought and wellbeing.

4. Accept yourself before your goal is reached.

Let me tell you something that I hope you already know. If you want happiness in life, you have to accept yourself, regardless of your size, shape, color or charisma. I've witnessed every type of motivation in people and do you know who is the most successful in their weight loss journey? The people that have already chosen to accept and love every single good and bad piece of themselves before their goal weight was ever reached.

So regardless of what you've tried to do in the past, accept yourself now and give yourself grace going forward. Do that and I guarantee you're going to experience much more success!

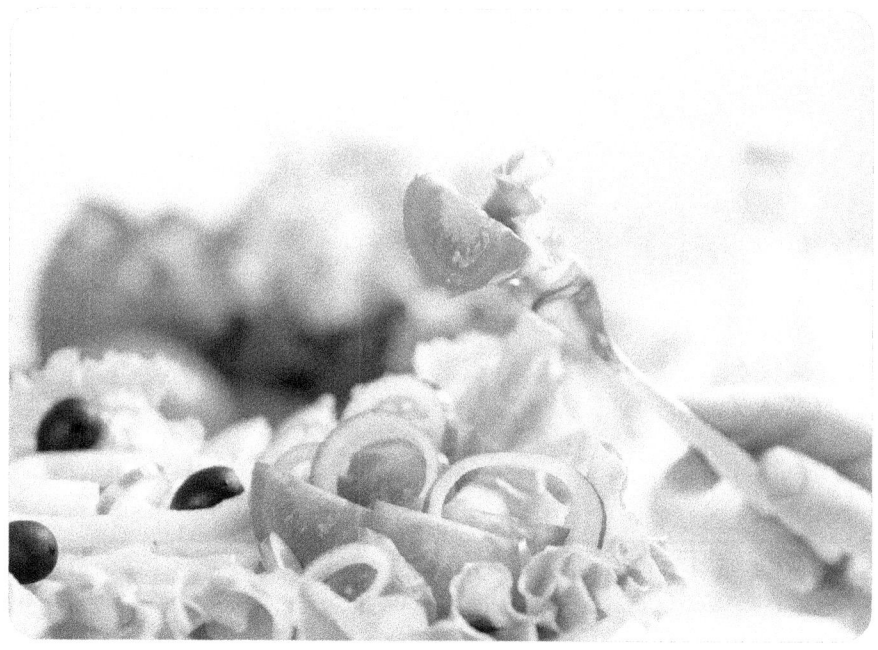

Chapter 5

LIVING OUT THE PACIFIC NORTHWEST LIFESTYLE

Well we're nearly at the end and I hope you've considered adopting this Pacific Northwest Lifestyle for yourself. Before we're through, let's recap a little bit.

THE 5 PRACTICES FOR LIVING A PACIFIC NORTHWEST LIFESTYLE

1. Food Has Flavor
2. Embrace Thy Outdoors
3. Live Leisurely
4. Mainly a Gatherer, Not a Hunter
5. Very Little Bags and Boxes

YOUR NEXT STEPS

We've talked about a plan that follows 5 simple practices. It's not complicated because I've done the research for you and boiled it down to what's going to give you the most improvement with the least effort. Lives today are busier than ever and the average person is bombarded with lies when it comes to health, hence the simplicity to help you get started right away.

You may have tried many approaches to improve your health in the past and may have even failed more times than you care to remember. Can this plan still work well for you? Yes. It's based off of the world's wisdom of what works well for

EVERYONE! Good health, bad health, young, old, busy, bored, male, female... I know it will work well for you too!

Once again...

Think back to what got you started into looking at your health in the first place? Why is living a healthier lifestyle important for you personally?

If you have your reasons in mind, then I challenge you to write down the 5 practices of The Pacific Northwest Lifestyle along with a to-do list of how to put them into practice in your own life.

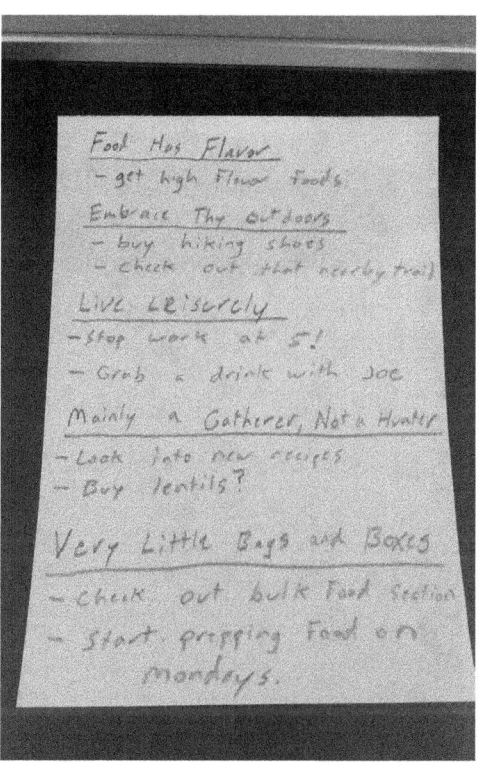

Then, pick a date in the future. Maybe a month from now, or maybe just a couple of weeks and make it your plan to put this lifestyle to work until that date. If you like where you end up, consider making this a permanent change for yourself as you live a fuller and more fulfilling healthy life.

Let's Make a Healthier Tomorrow – Asking a favor

Public health has suffered tremendously because we've moved away from basic principles that used to keep us healthy. There's widespread misinformation and it drives me crazy if you can't tell!

Millions of people will die unnecessary deaths because of large food corporation advertising and money-hungry marketers look at the obesity rate, as a business opportunity.

Well here is my favor to ask of you (it's actually a few flavors)...

- Stop describing food in terms of macronutrients (carbs, fat and protein)
- Don't listen to anyone using dreamy phrases such as: "fat burning", "cleansing", "getting ripped" or anything of the sort.
- Be your own health advocate and remember that food is medicine.

I'm pretty passionate about our current state of wellbeing if you can't tell and it pains me to hear of so much confusion around something that should be simple.

Just know that we eat whole foods (apples, peanut butter, lettuce, etc.). We don't eat just "carbs", "fats" or "proteins". In my humble opinion and experience, those who resort to using dreamy phrases like the ones above, or who talk about foods just as individual nutrients... these people are typically uneducated, deceptive individuals who are more focused on your attention and pocketbook than your wellbeing or prosperity.

Avoid them and look for unbiased answers to your health questions from those who truly want to help.

Okay, that is all. Be well my friends and thank you for investing attention into The Pacific Northwest Lifestyle!

Appendix A

GETTING STARTED GUIDE

■ *PAC NW Food Plan & Grocery List*
■ *20 meals Made with NW Style*

Pac NW Food Plan
(Grocery List and 1 Week of Meals Planned)

■ Beans (canned or dry) - Black Beans, Chickpeas, Roasted and Dried Chickpeas, White Beans, Red Lentils, Brown Lentils

■ Grains – Quinoa, Millet, Couscous, Popcorn, Rolled Oats, Brown Rice, Sprouted Bread, Sprouted Corn or Wheat Tortillas, Whole Wheat Spaghetti

■ Crackers – Flax and Rye

■ Nuts – Walnuts, Almonds, Pecans, Cashews, Peanut Butter, Almond Butter

■ Milks – Unsweetened Vanilla Soy Milk, Unsweetened Almond Milk

■ Seeds – Sunflower seeds, Pumpkin Seeds, Flaxseeds, Chia Seeds

■ Salad Ingredients – Kale, Lettuce, Red Cabbage, Green Cabbage, Spinach

■ Dried fruit – Raisins, Dates, Cranberries, Figs, Dried Apple Slices

■ Fruit – Banana, Berries (frozen are more inexpensive), Guava, Cranberry (fresh or canned sauce), Peaches, Apples, Oranges

■ Unsweetened Dried Coconut

■ Veggies – Jicama, Bell Pepper (red and green), Broccoli, Asparagus Corn – (fresh or frozen), Mushrooms (small white and Portabello) Cauliflower, Peas, Dried and Seasoned Peas, Cucumber, Olives, Zucchini, Tomato, Egg

Plant, Pumpkin (canned), Red Cabbage, Jalapenos, Tomato Soup, Onions (red and sweet) and at least 1 variety of cruciferous vegetable (broccoli, Brussels sprouts, collard greens, kale)

- Avocado
- Tofu – Hard and Soft varities
- Tempeh – Bacon strips
- Sweet Potato
- Squash
- Seasoning and Flavors – Balsamic Vinegar, Honey Mustard Dressing, Stevia or Errythritol for sweetness, Tahini Dressing, BBQ Sauce, Peanut Sauce, Nutritional Yeast, Cocoa Powder
- Hummus
- Salsa

20 Meals Made with Northwest Style

5 Breakfast Ideas

HOMEMADE GRANOLA CEREAL –

Combine:

- 1/4 cashews
- 1/2 cup dried dates chopped
- 2 tbsp pumpkin seeds

Top with:

- 1 cup unsweetened vanilla soy milk

Berry Smoothie –

Blend all ingredients until pureed:

- 1 cup almond milk
- 1/2 cup berries of choice
- 1 cup baby spinach
- 2 tbsp flaxseed
- 1/2 frozen banana chopped

Hot Quinoa Bowl –
Heat up the following ingredients in a microwave or enjoy cold:

- ½ cup cooked quinoa
- ½ cup unsweetened vanilla soy milk
- ¼ cup crushed walnuts
- ¼ cup chopped dates
- Top with: Cinnamon, ground cloves and Nutmeg

Sprouted Toast with Hummus –
- 2 slices sprouted bread toasted
- 4 tbsp of hummus as spread
- topped with stir fried mushrooms and onion slices

The REALLY Oregon Burrito –
- 1 large whole wheat tortilla
- wrapped with 1/2 avocado sliced
- 1/2 cup brown lentils, 2 tbsp salsa
- 1/2 cup black beans
- 2 tbsp low fat sour cream

5 Lunch Ideas

CRANBERRY AND ALMOND BUTTER SANDWICH –

Toast up 2 slices of sprouted bread.

Spread with 2 tbsp cranberry sauce on one slice and 2 tbsp almond butter on the other. Cut into two triangles. Just like Mom used to.

Cheesy" Tomato Soup & Rye Crackers –
Heat up 1 cup of Tomato Soup and sprinkle on top 1 tbsp of Nutritional Yeast. Stir into the soup until well combined. Have 3 Rye Crackers for dipping or crushing on top of soup. Whatever you fancy.

Evergreen as it Gets Apple Spinach Salad –
Mix together 1 cup Spinach, 1 chopped Celery stick, 1/4 cup of raw Sunflower Seeds, 1 Chopped Granny Smith Apple, 1/2 cup of Cucumber slices and drizzle with balsamic vinegar dressing.

Veggie sandwich –
Using Sandwich thin buns or 2 slices of sprouted toast, spread each side of bread with hummus, layer hot slices of firm tofu. Then top with roasted red tomatoes, red onion, lettuce and spicy mustard.

Spicy Red Lentil Soup –
Heat up 1 cup of Lentil Soup (homemade or canned, dice some roasted red peppers and add these in with salt, pepper, red pepper flakes, onion powder and garlic. Continue heating and stirring until all are well combined.

5 Dinner Ideas

5 Min Black Bean Burgers -

- 15 ounces black beans, drained and rinsed
- 2 tbsp ketchup
- 1 tbsp yellow mustard
- 1 tsp garlic powder

- 1 tsp onion powder
- 1 tbsp nutritional yeast
- 1/3 cup instant oats

In a mixing bowl, mash beans with a fork until about half the beans are squashed. In a mixing bowl, mash beans with a fork until about half the beans are squashed. Stir in condiments and spices until well combined. Then mix in oats. Divide into 4 thin patties.
Bake, grill or pan fry with a tiny bit of oil until crusty on each side.

Tip: Refrigerating for 30 min prior to cooking improves texture too.

Brown Rice and Mushroom Stir Fry –

Prepare 1 cup of brown rice in any way and place to the side. Slice 5 white button mushrooms and 1/2 small onion. Sautee these in a non-stick pan with 1/2 cup tomato sauce. Cook on medium heat until mushrooms are soft, stirring frequently. Then place over 1 cup brown rice.

Next mix together in a salad bowl 1/2 cup white beans, 1 cup spinach, 1/2 cup peas, 1/2 avocado sliced. Dress with honey mustard dressing.

Parmesan Tomato Zucchini Boats –

Cut 1 large zucchini in half and use a spoon to partially carve out the middles of the zucchini slices. Fill the insides with 1/2 cup brown lentils, diced tomatoes, basil and oregano. Sprinkle 2 tbsp of parmesan cheese on top. Bake in the oven at 350 until zucchini is totally soft.

Butternut Squash and Seitan Burrito –

Fill 1 whole wheat tortilla with sliced mushrooms, 1/2 cooked butternut squash, 2-3oz cooked seitan, 1/2 avocado sliced and 2 tbsp salsa. Wrap up and serve hot!

Rice Paper Veggie wraps with Peanut Sauce –

Take 2 brown rice papers and soak till soft. Then spread on plate, filling with 1 cup finely chopped broccoli, 1/2 cup chickpeas, 1/2 cup shredded cabbage,

1/2 cup grated carrots and cucumber slices. Roll up tightly and dip into 2 tbsp peanut sauce.

Four Bean Salad —

Mix together in large bowl 1 cup Kidney Beans, 1 cup White Beans, 1 cup Green Beans and 1 cup Brown Lentils (crock pot or canned). Top with 1/4 cup diced onions, 2 tbsp honey mustard, 1 tbsp olive oil and balsamic vinegar. Mix well. Refrigerate and serve cool for a quick filling side.

5 Snack Ideas

5 Minute No Bake Protein Bars -

- 1/2 banana mashed
- 6 Tbsp natural peanut butter (or almond butter)
- 1 scoop Plant Protein Powder (pea, soy or brown rice preferred)
- 1/3 cup ground flaxseed
- 1/2 - 2 Tbsp almond milk (if needed for texture)

Mix the following ingredients in a bowl in the order listed. Aim for a sticky consistency that can be formed into thin bars.

Spread the mixture on a pan and cut into 5 delicious on-the-go bars.

Roasted, Sweet Chickpeas -

Using 1 15 oz can of chickpeas, spread the peas out on a paper towel and pat dry (it helps to let them air dry for a little bit too). The drier they are, the more you'll be able to flavor them later on!

Once dry, collect them in a large bowl and drizzle with 1 tbsp olive oil.

Cook in the oven at 375 until crispy (usually around 45 min). Lastly, sprinkle with 1 tsp cinnamon, 1/8 tsp nutmeg, 1/8 tsp stevia and 1/8 tsp sea salt.

Can be made in large batches too!

Homemade Trailmix -

This is a simple one. Mix together 1 cup low-fat granola cereal, 1/2 cup chopped dates, 1/2 cup sunflower seeds and 2 tbsp unsweetened shredded coconut. Store in an airtight container and use as an on-the-go snack.

Chocolate Pumpkin Cookies -

- 1/2 cup peanut butter
- 1/2 cup rolled oats
- 1/2 cup unsweetened cocoa powder
- 1/4 teaspoon fine sea salt
- 3/4 cup pumpkin purée
- 1/2 cup unsalted natural creamy peanut butter
- 2 teaspoons pure vanilla extract
- 1 cup finely chopped pitted dates (6 ounces whole dates)

Mix all dry ingredients in a bowl and sift together. Then, in a separate bowl, combine peanut butter, pumpkin puree, vanilla and chopped dates. Mix together using a food processor or electric mixer. Then combine with the dry ingredients just until mixed.

Place 2 tbsp size balls of dough onto pan and bake at 350 degrees just until edges are browned.

The BEST 2 Ingredient Ice Cream -

The trick to this is freezing bananas ahead of time (always a good idea to keep a stash of frozen bananas in the freezer for smoothies too).

Take 1 frozen banana and chop it into ½ slices. Add to blender and top with 2 tbsp peanut butter. Blend together for an ice cream consistency and add 1-2 tbsp almond milk if needed for blending.

Optional Add ons: Vanilla extract, cinnamon, stevia, dates, cocoa powder.

REFERENCES

1. Interactive Atlas of Heart Disease and Stroke." Maps. Centers for Disease Control and Prevention, n.d. Web. 14 Jan. 2015.

2. Interactive Atlas of Heart Disease and Stroke." Maps. Centers for Disease Control and Prevention, n.d. Web. 14 Jan. 2015.

3. A. Britton, M.G. Marmot, & M. Shipley. Who benefits most from the cardioprotective properties of alcohol consumption—health freaks or couch potatoes. J Epidemiol Community Health, 62(10):905-908, 2008.

4. Public Health Agency of Canada. (2009). Tracking Heart Disease and Stroke in Canada, 2009. Retrieved from: http://www.phac-aspc.gc.ca/publicat/2009/cvd-avc/pdf/cvd-avs-2009-eng.pdf

5. Hug, Stella-Maria, et al. "Restorative qualities of indoor and outdoor exercise settings as predictors of exercise frequency." Health & Place 15.4 (2009): 971-980.

6. Thompson Coon, J., et al. "Does participating in physical activity in outdoor natural environments have a greater effect on physical and mental wellbeing than physical activity indoors? A systematic review." Environmental science & technology 45.5 (2011): 1761-1772.

7. Shiota, Masatoshi, Masamichi Sudou, and Masamitsu Ohshima. "Using outdoor exercise to decrease jet lag in airline crewmembers." Aviation, space, and environmental medicine 67.12 (1996): 1155-1160.

8. Vergnaud AC, Norat T, Romaguera D, Mouw T, May AM, Travier N, Luan J, Wareham N, Slimani N, Rinaldi S, Couto E, Clavel-Chapelon F, Boutron-Ruault MC, Cottet V, Palli D, Agnoli C, Panico S, Tumino R, Vineis P, Agudo A, Rodriguez L, Sanchez MJ, Amiano P, Barricarte A, Huerta JM, Key TJ, Spencer EA, Bueno-de-Mesquita B, Büchner FL, Orfanos P, Naska

www.ingramcontent.com/pod-product-compliance
Lightning Source LLC
Chambersburg PA
CBHW060105300526
45788CB00015B/1895